Food Essentials
for the Busy Professional

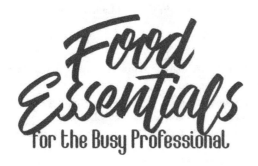

Food Essentials
for the Busy Professional

LAUREN POWELL, MD
The Culinary Doctor

purposely
created
PUBLISHING

FOOD ESSENTIALS FOR THE BUSY PROFESSIONAL

Published by Purposely Created Publishing Group™

Printed in the United States of America

ISBN: 978-1-64484-036-8

Disclaimer

This book is for informational and educational purposes only and should not be misconstrued as official medical advice. This book is not intended to be a substitute for professional medical advice, diagnosis, or treatment. Always seek the advice of your physician or other qualified health providers with any questions you may have regarding a medical condition or with changing your dietary habits. Never disregard professional medical advice or delay in seeking it because of something you have read or seen in this book.

Dedication

First, I want to take a few lines of this book to express gratitude. To Jesus Christ, my Lord and Savior who knew me before I was thought of and whose love sustains me in my most challenging moments, I am thankful for the opportunity to live the life You have blessed me to live. My prayer is that my life brings You honor.

To my husband, my love, my best friend, and the one who makes my heart flutter: I'm so unconditionally thankful to share this life on earth with you. Thank you for your support, encouragement, and for your love.

To my momma and papa whose shoulders I stand on: I can never thank you enough or repay you for all you've done for me. All I want to do is make you proud.

To all my girlfriends, my village: Thanks for celebrating the triumphs with me and encouraging me through the challenges. You bring me so much joy. I love you and thank you for your support.

To my coaches, Dr. Drai and Dr. Toni Haley, thank you for pushing me beyond my limits. Thank you for dreaming big for me when I could not dream big for myself. Thank you to my mentor, Dr. Bonnie Simpson Mason, for living your life in a way that pushes me to be better for all of those around me. Thank you for holding my hand and for being, hands down, the best hype woman ever. I love you all.

This book is dedicated to every woman who desires to be the change she wishes to see. We wear many hats. Some call us friend, sister, daughter, mother, wife, aunt, niece, grandmother, and to others we are community leaders, colleagues, and executives. Growing up and to this day, I believed that my mother was capable of doing the impossible and solving all problems. I think all daughters see their mothers this way.

The health status of the black community continues to be poor. Let's end that. Let's decide as women that no one in our family will be obese, suffer from heart disease, have diabetes, or have their life significantly changed because of a stroke. Let's teach our family health-promoting lifestyle behaviors, healthy food and cooking techniques, and change generational patterns of disease. Yes, the task is great, but we are women, and we were created to exceed greatness.

Table of Contents

Foreword

for the Culinary Doctor

It is important for each one of us to be able to identify and be thankful for people in our lives who are true blessings.

Dr. Lauren Powell is one of those true blessings in the lives of her patients, her family, friends and for me, personally. In her, you will find one of the most genuine, whip smart, beautiful and sincerely helpful individuals on the planet. Her attributes don't stop there. She's creative, resourceful and industrious, always seeking to provide new information in a way that improves the lives of the people around her and her patients, from the inside out.

Dr. Lauren Powell, the Culinary Doctor, will nourish you through food and through inspiration, because that's who she is and that's her passion, and I truly look forward to taking in, literally and figuratively, all that Dr. Lauren has to offer.

I'm sure as you read through her food principles and tips, for yourself and your family, that you will also digest:

~All of the love that she provides in each chapter

~All of the smiles she pours into each dish that she makes

~And all of the enthusiasm for life that she emanates daily through healthy living

Why? Because Dr. Lauren Powell is as a beacon of light and a shining example of what's possible for all of us, and we thank God for that. She is answering the call to educate us on how to live, eat, and be better.

So, please share as you enjoy Dr. Lauren Powell, the Culinary Doctor's first book of many, as well as her blogs, video courses, and TV appearances.

As members of her global "Culinary Doctor Fan Club," we wish her the very best that life has to offer, because that is what she giving to us—one recipe at a time.

Bon appétit and blessings!

Dr. Bonnie Mason

Introduction

My name is Dr. Lauren Powell, and I am a board-certified family medicine physician and culinary medicine specialist. I help individuals and families prevent and cure disease through food. Through my online programs, books, and live events, I teach them healthy cooking techniques that they can use to optimize their health and end generational patterns of chronic disease.

I grew up in the suburbs outside of Detroit. My family owned drycleaners. Everyone in the family, at some point in their life, worked at the drycleaners. Grandma was the seamstress, my cousins worked with the customers, several of my aunts and uncles worked at the cleaners at various times throughout their lives, and my brother and I started tagging clothes on Saturday when we were seven and eight years old. The dry cleaning business was all I knew.

When I was in the 8th grade, we were given an assignment to write a story with an accompanying illustration of what we wanted to be when we grow up. I did not hesitate. I knew when I grew up, I would work at a drycleaners like my parents. I remember

1

writing that on my paper and then looking at the other students' work. No one else had written that they wanted to work at a drycleaners. The most popular girl in the school wrote that she wanted to be a pediatrician. I thought since she was smart, this must be a good idea. I went home from school that day and told my parents I was going to become a doctor. My parents had not graduated from college and were from very humble beginnings, so they were surprised at my statement but still encouraged me.

Becoming a doctor became my plan, and I stuck to it. I graduated from high school and attended the University of Detroit Mercy on a full academic scholarship. I graduated cum laude with a bachelor's degree in chemistry and a minor in business administration. I then went on to medical school at Wayne State University. I did very well there and decided that I wanted to be a family medicine doctor. I attended Halifax Health Family Medicine Residency in Daytona Beach, Florida, one of the top family medicine residency programs in the country. I was very interested in research and presented several publications on both local and national platforms. During my last year of residency, I was selected by my peers and supervising physicians to serve as chief resident.

While residency was an exciting and fulfilling time, it was also very demanding. As a senior resident, it was our responsibility to take thirty-hour call. This means we would start the day at 7 a.m., work all day and overnight, and then leave around 11 a.m. the next day. It was demanding, and the nights could be very stressful. It became part of my routine that when I finished my call shift in the afternoon, I would get in my convertible with the top down to make up for the past 30 hours of no fresh air or sunlight. It was also part of my routine to call my dad on my drive home to keep me awake on my drive.

One Saturday morning, I called my dad rambling on about the challenging cases I had overnight. Then I noticed my father wasn't responding as much as he regularly would. When he would speak, his speech was extremely muffled and difficult to understand. I asked what was wrong and he told me that he wasn't sure; he had just woken up having a hard time saying the words he was thinking. I immediately knew my father was having stroke. I instructed him to hang up the phone and drive to the hospital. He told me he thought he was just tired and needed to finish cleaning the clothes and making the deliveries. I told my father very sternly that he could either drive to the nearest hospital or that

I would call 911. He agreed to drive to the hospital. I called my mother and told her that her husband was having a stroke and to get to the hospital. In the ER, my father put the phone on speaker. I heard him answer the ER physician's questions. When he asked, "What brings you in today?" My father replied in a very hard to comprehend way, "I'm having a hard time speaking and can't move the right side of my body." Urgently, my father was taken back for imaging and testing. They discovered that my father had suffered a stroke, and he remained in the hospital for several days.

While admitted, he was also diagnosed with elevated blood pressure, diabetes, and elevated cholesterol. I felt horrible. I was his daughter and a doctor, and I felt like I had not done a good job of educating and explaining to him how the food he was putting in his body was affecting his health. I knew that his stroke was directly related to his poor diet.

African-American adults are one and a half times more likely than Caucasian adults to be obese. According to the American Heart Association, African Americans carry a higher burden of cardiovascular disease compared to white Americans[1].

---

1 https://newsroom.heart.org/news/african-americans-live-shorter-lives-due-to-heart-disease-and-stroke

Additionally, African Americans are twice as likely to be diagnosed with diabetes. Obesity, heart disease, and diabetes are all preventable diseases[2]. Studies have consistently shown the role that a poor diet plays in these preventable diseases, and oftentimes these diseases are seen in multiple generations of the same family because of similar lifestyle, dietary, and cooking habits. Addressing these health disparities begins by educating minorities about the value and role of nutrition in living healthier lives.

I have devoted a significant amount of time educating myself about the role of food and nutrition in health, so that I would have the skills to not only change my lifestyle and educate my family members, but to also educate and empower my patients. I have become committed to teaching others, particularly in the African-American community, how to optimize their health, prevent chronic disease, and eliminate generational conditions through healthy cooking techniques and meals. Some people leave their family and community money, property, and heirlooms. I am leaving a legacy of good health and a disease-free life.

---

2 https://minorityhealth.hhs.gov/omh/browse.aspx?lvl=4&lvlid=18

Chapter 1

Food & Your Purpose

Do you believe that living your best life is directly related to your health? Do you believe that your health is directly related to the food you put inside your body? I'm going to help you and say that what you put in your body is DIRECTLY related to your health, and if your health is not optimized, you cannot live your God-given purpose. Think about it: when you have a cold, you're not at your best. The same is true when you have poor energy, fatigue, inability to sleep, are overweight, and suffering from medical issues; you're simply not at your best. The difference between the conditions I just named and a cold is we get used to suffering with those conditions and don't even realize we aren't functioning at our highest potential (until we fix our nutrition and no longer have those problems).

Your health is just that: it's your health. Oftentimes my patients try to put their health in my hands. As their physician, my role is not to tell them what to do. My role is to be a resource, providing the latest in evidence-based medical knowledge and assisting the client in helping to make a decision that is best for them. Therefore, I encourage my patients to cook and learn about how food affects their health and can be used to prevent and cure disease. If a patient is on medication, they are dependent on me. But if a patient is able to manage their disease with proper nutrition, they are in complete control of their health. I'm just the cheerleader.

There's no quick fix to a healthy lifestyle. As you read this book and reflect on changes you want to make in your life, I challenge you to ask yourself with regards to any change, "Can I maintain this for the rest of my life?" We are not trying to make 30-day, 4-month, or one-year changes. The goal is sustainable lifestyle changes that we can maintain for our whole life. After all, we want to be healthy for our entire lives, not just for a short period of it.

We can't talk about a healthy lifestyle and nutrition without a mention about exercise. The goal of exercise is 150 minutes of activity a week. You can divide those minutes up how you like. Maybe

20 minutes in the morning, 30 minutes during your lunch break, and 15 minutes after work. I find that by thinking about exercise in terms of minutes makes it seem less overwhelming and gives more flexibility. Additionally, find something that you enjoy. If you don't like running, don't buy a treadmill. Think of a realistic option for you. Instead, try different forms of exercise: Zumba, step aerobics, HIT, swimming, spinning, barre, kickboxing, the list goes on and on. If it's something you enjoy, you're more likely to do it.

Finally, in addition to loving your exercise, you should love the food you're consuming. If you're going to be upset about only eating vegetables, then don't do it. If you're going to be upset that you can't eat any bread, then that should not be a principle of your nutrition. I am excited about the food that I put in my body. I am primarily a vegetarian and eat fish on some occasions. I love what I eat and don't feel like I'm missing out on anything. I understand that the food I'm putting in my body is fueling my body, so it can function at its optimum. And I know that some foods don't allow me to feel my best, so I am okay with not consuming those items.

Chapter 2

Food & Disease

D id you know that there are several medical conditions that have been directly linked to certain
foods? I am often surprised when I talk to a patient
who has had hypertension for over ten years, and
no one has ever talked to them about their salt con-
tent. Or women who have battled breast cancer on
multiple occasions who have never been counseled
about the role of diet in preventing inflammation in
the body. It is true that diabetes, obesity, high cholesterol, high blood pressure, and some cancers are
directly linked to diet, and are therefore considered
preventable diseases.

Certain conditions run in families. For instance,
multiple family members can be overweight or take
medication for their elevated blood pressure or diabetes. While genetics do play a role in health, what
places a larger role, I believe, are social and lifestyle
factors. Certain diseases run in a family because

everyone in that family is cooking and eating the same way. Cooking techniques are often passed down. That's why I love teaching about cooking so much, because I know when I empower someone with culinary skills, it's not just going to improve their health but the health of their parents, children, and anyone who comes after them.

If you have elevated blood pressure, there is a basic principle you must follow. You must WATCH YOUR SALT. Often when I make this statement to my patients, the first thing they say is, "Doc, I don't add any salt to my food." I remind them that it's not just about the salt shaker on the counter. It's about the seasonings that we cook with that contain salt, the dressings we use, the gravy, the sauces like soy and siracha that we can't get enough of, the canned soups and vegetables, and the deli and breakfast meat that we purchase. All of these items contain an abundance of salt, and when consumed on a regular basis can worsen your blood pressure or make it hard to control.

Diabetes is also a disease largely influenced by diet. I find that my patients are often on one of two ends of the spectrum. Either they are giving no consideration to what they put in their body and come to my office with a bag of Skittles, or they are so severely restricting their diet that they are malnourished. Eating to effectively manage or prevent diabetes is about minimizing sugar and simple carbohydrate consumption and increasing fiber and protein. I find that one of the greatest challenges when it comes to sugar consumption are the beverages. The juices, Starbucks beverages, energy drinks, and the soda pops often contain a lot of sugar that we are completely unaware of. Watch out for these items.

While we are talking health and disease, I also wanted to talk briefly about our skin health. Starting in middle school, and then worsening in college, I suffered from acne. In addition to the breakouts, my acne left hyperpigmented scars on my forehead, chin, and cheeks. I finally sought medical attention in college and was on three different prescriptions to manage it. After finishing medical school and making significant dietary changes, my skin significantly improved and I stopped taking all the acne medications. My friends, peers, and patients often ask me my skin care routine, and I tell them very simply, "I eat my way to clear skin and healthy hair." There's a reason why acne occurs mostly in populations that follow a Western diet. Here are some basic tips that I follow:

- Avoid high saturated fat, which stimulates hormones to produce more sebum (oil).

- The more unprocessed your diet, the better. That means more fruits and vegetables and less drive-throughs and prepackaged snacks.

- Eat foods rich in vitamin A and zinc. You don't need supplements. Your body absorbs these nutrients better from the source than a pill. My favorite source of vitamin A is kale, and I get plenty of zinc from all the beans I eat!

- Your body and skin love water! In college I lived off lemonade and Red Bull. Now, it's one cup of coffee in the morning then water for the rest of the day.

- If you do nothing else, make sure you wear a daily moisturizer with SPF to protect your skin from sun damage.

Chapter 3

Principles I Live By

I have created a list of six food principles that I live by. They are the principles I share with every audience that I speak with. I use these principles in an effort to keep things simple yet all-encompassing.

First principle: Plants

Eat more plants and eat them often. The studies are definitive. Those who eat more plants live healthier, longer lives. Not every meal has to have meat. If you're a meat lover and gotta have a slab of meat on your place for breakfast, lunch, and dinner, I'm not asking you to become a vegan tomorrow. I'm challenging you to make small changes. For example, start with one specific meal, like breakfast, that does not contain meat. Or maybe choose one day a week, like a meatless Monday. Replace that meat with a plant-based protein or high fiber legumes.

Second principle: Cooking

We have to cook our food because that is the only way we can control what's in the food we are consuming. I have a few colleagues who hate cooking. I mean just the thought of going into their kitchen gives them palpitations. I think sometimes we put way too much pressure on ourselves. Pressure to make the perfect meal that's fancy and complex. I encouraged one of my friends who felt this exact way to start just by making sides and purchasing a rotisserie chicken from her local grocery store. You should've seen the sigh of relief when I offered her this suggestion. A half home-cooked meal is better than a complete carryout.

Third principle: Ingredients

Always look at the ingredients of the food you purchase. Ideally, you want to recognize all the ingredients. You want the food you purchase to have less than five ingredients. Remember, ingredients are listed from their highest component to lowest. So if sugar or salt is listed as the first ingredient, watch out.

Fourth principle: Beverages

This will be covered in more detail later, but I always suggest three main beverages in your life: number one is water. This is what you should be consuming in greatest amount. Next, is red wine and black coffee—both of which, when consumed in moderation, have a health benefit.

Fourth principle: Mindful eating

This topic is so huge, there is an entire chapter dedicated to this. Practicing mindful eating is what helps us appreciate our food and not overeat.

Fifth principle: Being mindful of the environment

My friends all know that I love the orangutans, I love the dolphins and sea lions, and I want my kids to grow up seeing wildlife in their natural habitat. If we can each do our part, by being responsible for ourselves and the products we use, we can preserve our wonderful world for future generations. Avoid plastic; grocery shop using reusable bags. Use recycled plates, bring your travel mug to the coffee shop instead of using the paper ones, use reusable straws, and walk when you can to help air pollution. Shop locally and pick foods that are in season, as they are less likely being shipped from other countries. I'm all about not overeating and don't believe in "eat until your plate is clean." Instead, try to consider portions before you cook. For instance, when I make garlic bread for my husband and me, I only make one piece per person, because that is a serving size. If I make more, we may overeat or waste food. If you can't finish your plate, bring it for lunch the next day, or use the leftovers to create a new dish. I often bring leftovers to work and share it with my staff; they are always so happy and grateful.

Chapter 4

Mindful Eating

This is one of my favorite topics. Mindful eating entails remaining in the present moment and fully experiencing your food. When we don't practice mindfulness while eating, we overeat, do not get to fully experience the flavors of our food, and consume our food quickly causing gastrointestinal upset. I am going to detail five ways that you and your family can practice mindful eating below:

1. Always begin your meal with a moment of gratitude. Acknowledge how blessed and fortunate you are to be able to eat and enjoy the food that you have. Pray for those who are less fortunate and may be going throughout their day hungry, and be thankful for those that you get to enjoy your meal with.

2. Your meals should be enjoyed at the dinner table without distractions. This means you

should not be watching TV, listening to a podcast, talking on the phone, or engaging in any other activities that would distract you from being fully present with your meal. I strongly suggest the 'no cell phone at the dinner table' rule. In homes with adults and teenagers, commit to everyone putting their phones on top of the refrigerator until after dinner is complete. Although this will be challenging initially, it will soon become routine and a time to look forward to without distractions.

3. Chew your food. No, really, chew it. Don't inhale it and do not swallow it whole. Chew soft food approximately 5-10 times, and the harder, more fibrous food up to 30 times. While chewing your food, think about and acknowledge the taste, the flavor, and the texture. Enjoy how the seasonings and herbs work together to create such a dynamic taste. Acknowledge this for yourself and share it with guests. Trust me, you'll enjoy it, and whoever prepared the food will enjoy it as well.

4. Eat your food on a plate. We will talk more at length about this when we get to the section on portion control, but it is very important to

put your food on a plate and not eat out of the bag, carton, or box the food may have come in. For instance, a serving size of potato chips is usually about 11 chips. If I gave you a whole bag, do you think you would just eat 11 chips? Probably not. But if you counted out 11 chips and put them on a plate, you are more likely to stay within the serving size. Oftentimes when we eat out of a bag, we eat mindlessly and are not cued that we should stop eating until we reach the end of the bag, not realizing we should've stopped about 25 chips ago.

5. Lastly, and most important, ask yourself while eating, "How hungry am I?" The hunger scale is from 1-10—1 being starving and feeling like you're going to pass out and 10 being so full you feel uncomfortable like you want to vomit. It is important while you are eating, that you constantly ask yourself how hungry you are. You don't want to be too hungry, but you also don't want to be too full. I try to stay between a level 3 (hungry, but not uncomfortable) and then eat until I am at a level 6-7 (filled up but comfortable). You don't necessarily want to just eat until all the food is off

of your plate because oftentimes, especially when it comes to restaurant food, that means overeating. Gone are the days of eating until your plate is clean. If you're full, don't force yourself to finish the food. Instead, wrap up the leftovers for lunch or to create another dish with.

Chapter 5

Balance

A healthy lifestyle is just that, it's a lifestyle. This is not a quick fix. The goal is to create sustainable lifestyle changes. With that being said, we have to be realistic. So I want to give you a few concepts that are crucial to your healthy lifestyle.

First, the cheat meal. Now I said cheat meal. I did not say cheat day, cheat weekend, or cheat week. Once a week, I want you to plan for a meal that you will enjoy. For me, it's Friday date night with my husband. I know that on Friday we will go to a nice restaurant, and I anticipate the appetizer we will share, the one cocktail I will have, and the entree of my choice. I enjoy the meal without guilt, and on Saturday morning it's right back to my routine. Cheat meals are important because they allow you to enjoy special events and ensure that you are not missing out. What's crucial here is that it's a cheat MEAL, not day. A whole day of eating however you want can set you back weeks. After you worked hard all week with your exercise and good nutrition, who wants to waste all that hard work?

Second, understand and accept that some foods just can't be made healthy. I don't care what anyone says, vegan mac and cheese does not taste as good as my momma's mac and cheese she makes for Christmas. Instead of making unhealthy things healthy, just enjoy healthy things. So I can't eat mac and cheese on a regular basis. That's okay, because on Christmas I'm smashing it. Instead of trying to make your tofu into a steak, just enjoy things that are healthy and tasty in their natural state. Experiment with different vegetables and legumes. Bake a type of fish you've never made before. Try some new seasonings to spice up your vegetables. The possibilities are endless.

Lastly: plan. If you're going on vacation, attending a wedding, or doing anything that takes you off your routine, you have to plan. You can't just go into these type of events or away from home for a week and think things will just fall into place. It takes me three months to lose 10 pounds, and I can gain 10 pounds in one weekend by recklessly eating and drinking. Seriously, I've done it. And whenever I return from that cruise or conference and step on the scale, I'm so upset with myself. I went on these trips with no plan, ate without boundaries, and all my hard work was reversed in five days. It's never worth it, trust me. Enjoy the trip and the time away from home, but plan for that. Plan your meals, snacks, alcohol consumption, and exercise. See my chapter on travel for the details.

Chapter 6

Dietary Recommendations

The issue with many fad diets is the primary focus is usually on weight loss as opposed to health optimization. I want to provide you with some basic dietary fundamentals and recommend some dietary patterns. My goal for you as you embark on your journey to optimal health is that you continue to evolve in your culinary skills and broaden your dietary interest.

The Mediterranean Diet

When patients simply don't know what to eat, I find it works best to discuss the Mediterranean diet and its principles. When I use the word diet, I am referring to a way of eating, not a short-term weight loss plan. What I like most about the Mediterranean diet is that it is broad, meaning not super restrictive, and it's easy to follow. According to the American Family Physicians, the data and research provides strong evidence that when the Mediterranean diet is followed consistently, it:

- prevents diabetes type 2

- prevents age-related cognitive decline

- prevents heart disease

- can effectively be used to treat obesity

- decreases risk of cancer

- decreases risk of premature death

That's huge. I find the best way to describe this diet is utilizing their pyramid.

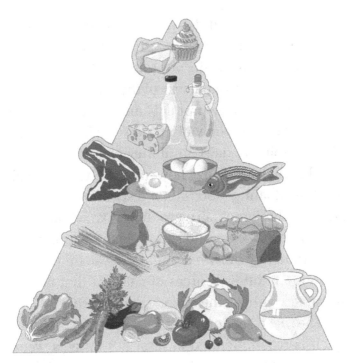

Figure 1.

Let's start at the top. The top of the triangle is the smallest section, meaning these are things we should eat very little of. For my patients who are unwilling to give up the red meat, I encourage them to limit the red meat and sweets for special occasions.

The next section is the eggs, poultry, and fermented dairy like cheese and yogurt. The Mediterranean diet does not support the consumption of milk, only fermented dairy. I support this for multiple reasons. First, many African Americans are lactose intolerant or do not tolerate dairy. Studies have shown up to 70 percent of the population cannot fully digest dairy products due to deficiency in the gene lactase. Many often don't realize their inability to tolerate dairy until they eliminate it from their diet then recognize how much better they feel, with less bloating, abdominal discomfort, and gas. Additionally, some dairy products, like whole milk, contain added sugar and saturated fat. I know what you're thinking: but what about the calcium? There are so many other sources of calcium that can be consumed without the added fat and carbs.

The next section refers to fish and seafood, which is recommended at least 2-3 times a week. For the Mediterranean diet, seafood is the main animal protein. I recommend my patients diversify and try different types of fish so that they are getting a varied nutrient profile.

The next section is the largest food section, and that is because it's where you should be getting most of your calories from. Each meal should contain a mixture of fruit, vegetables, and legumes. Olive oil is the cooking oil of choice, as it contains a large amount of monounsaturated fatty acids and antioxidants, which have been shown to have a health benefit. Other important food items in this section are your spices and herbs to season your food, nuts, seeds, and whole grains. These items should take up at least half of your plate.

At the bottom of the pyramid are general healthy lifestyle principles, like eating together as a family and living an active lifestyle. The Mediterranean diet encourages water as the main beverage with consumption of wine in moderation.

The Dietary Approaches to Stop Hypertension

The Dietary Approaches to Stop Hypertension, also known as the DASH diet, is usually where I start with my patients who have elevated blood pressure. If my patient's blood pressure is greater than 130/80, they can expect my talk about the DASH diet to ensue. This diet's primary focus is minimizing salt consumption. The recommended daily amount of salt is 2300 mg a day, although many people have consumed their daily allowance before lunch. The DASH diet is simple— avoid foods with high sodium: canned soups and vegetables, prepacked sauces and gravy, deli meat, and cheese, and eat more foods with little to no sodium like fresh fruits and vegetables, whole grains, and herbs and spices.

Chapter 7

Just Tell Me What to Eat

(Reference: American Family Physicians, June 1, 218, volume 97, 11 " Diets for Health: Goals and Guidelines")

I think the most common question I get from my patients with regards to food and diet is, "Doc, I just don't know what to eat." And I completely understand what they're saying. It can be confusing at times. Between the media, books, and news, people are very confused about what to put in their body. Do I eat meat, do I not eat meat? Do I drink milk or no? What about carbs? Are they all bad? Should I completely avoid sugar? It's hard sometimes just to know where to start and what to eat and what not to eat.

I think it's vital to understand all the different food groups and the role that they play. Anytime someone tells me they are planning on removing a food group from their diet, I ask what they plan on replacing it with. If you're going to stop eating fat, but then replace those calories with calories from carbohydrates, this may not be consistent with your health goal of losing inches around your waist. I'm also not a fan of making dietary changes that are for short periods of time. Again, this is about lifestyle and establishing good habits. We are not trying to live our best life for just 30 days but rather for our entire future.

Eat more plants. It is very simple, and the studies have been very clear: the more plants in your diet, the better the diet. The goal is a minimum of nine (9) servings of vegetables a day. For some, that may seem like a lot, and it does if you're waiting until dinner time to have your vegetables. Incorporate vegetables in every meal. When my husband and I got married, I would pack his lunch for work. Whatever the meal was, I always packed a container of vegetables to go along with it. One day he asked me why he had to have vegetables with every meal, why couldn't he just have spaghetti. I had to remind him that not only was I the wife, which means I'm all knowing, I'm a doctor, too, and you do in fact need to have vegetables with every meal. Increase your daily fruit and vegetable consumption, and you'll decrease your risk of diabetes, obesity, cancer, heart disease, and stroke.

Not all fats are created equal.

There are good fats and bad fats. We cannot compare the fat in an avocado to the fat in ham. Let's talk about the three main types of fats: trans fat, saturated fat, and unsaturated fat.

Trans fat

Trans fats are the worse. This is the type of fat that's found in highly processed food. Trans fats occur when an unsaturated fat is converted into a saturated fat in order to prolong the shelf life of a product. These types of fats are naughty because they increase your LDL (bad cholesterol) and lower your HDL (good cholesterol). Examples include margarine, doughnuts (sorry), and some frozen pizza. Always, always, always say no to trans fat.

Saturated fat

Saturated fat usually comes from animal products. Saturated fat from animal sources have been shown to have a negative effect on health, increasing the risk of coronary artery disease. Saturated fat from plant sources include olive oil, avocados, and flax seeds. Animal sources of saturated fat include meat from cows and pigs.

Unsaturated fat

Unsaturated fat, known as the "good" fat, is divided into two categories: monounsaturated and polyunsaturated fatty acids, more affectionately known as the MUFAs and the PUFAs. Polyunsaturated fatty acids are then divided into two types: omega 3 and omega 6. Sources of monounsaturated fatty acids are our oils—canola oil, sesame oil, and peanut butter to name a few. These types of fats have been shown to have a health benefit, but they still need to be consumed in moderation because of the calories. Sources of omega 3 fatty acids include wild fish and nuts. Omega 3 fatty acids have been shows to be beneficial for symptoms of depression, bipolar, and mild cognitive impairment. Sources of omega 6 fatty acids include avocados, almonds, and sunflower seeds. Omega 6 fatty acids are important in regulating blood pressure and for immune function. While both omega 6 and omega 3 fatty acids have health benefits, it is important to note that the American diet tends to contain more omega 6 fatty acids. An uneven ratio, or having a high amount of omega 6 fatty acids in comparison to omega 3 fatty acids, causes inflammation in the body which can cause adverse effects in the body. So focus on increasing your omega 3 fatty acids and your monounsaturated fatty acids, considering most people are getting enough omega 6 fatty acids.

Legumes

More beans, please. Another word for beans are legumes. This food group is extremely important because of the health benefits it provides. Beans have a high source of fiber. That's crucial because fiber is what helps you have healthy bowel movements, keeps you full, decreases the risk of heart disease and stroke, and decreases your risk of colon cancer. Additionally, beans are a great protein source. For those who do not eat meat, this is a great source of protein. The recommended portion is four servings in a week. I essentially try to incorporate legumes in at least one of my meals a day.

Whole grains

The power of whole grains. Just like all fats are not created equal, all carbohydrates are not created equal. Grains are healthy, but what happens in their processing to be stored on grocery store shelves is that all the nutritious components are removed. It's essentially comparing white rice, which is extremely processed, to brown or wild rice, which is very minimally processed. It takes longer to make those unprocessed grains, but they are more beneficial to your health. The USDA recommends eating 1.5-3 cups of grains per day, with at least half of these being from whole grains. I recommend that at least 70 percent of these be from whole grains.

Tea

Just say no to sweet tea. I mean a hard no. Herbal tea is great. Green tea with lemon and honey is great, too. But there's just no way around it; there is absolutely no health benefit to sweet tea. I always ask my patients, would you rather get your calories from food or through a straw?

Chapter 8

Serving Sizes

There are two factors to a healthy lifestyle when it comes to food: it's what you're putting in your body and how much. There is a such thing as too much of a good thing. Sometimes my husband thinks just because the chips are organic with minimal ingredients and low calories that he can eat as many as he wants. This is just not true. Calories and macronutrients add up. So you must always be mindful of the serving size of every single thing you eat. Now for food that comes in a bag or box, it may be easy to tell what the serving size it by reading the nutrition label, but it may be more difficult for items that are not prepacked. I have some tips for you!

- If you're having some nuts for a snack, you should eat no more than a handful. So this will different for a man with larger hands than it will for a petite female. That makes sense.

- For any kind of nut butter (peanut butter, almond butter, etc.), a serving size should be no bigger than a golf ball.

- For your legumes, think about a baseball. So for a meal, the beans on your plate should be no larger than a baseball.

- With meat, let's keep it simple. Think about a deck of cards. This is the approximate size of your portion of meat for a meal, if you are eating meat.

Next, I would like to discuss serving sizes for beverages. Your main beverage, or beverage of choice, should be water. Obviously, water over any beverage is best, and if you have access to various types of water, alkaline is best, artesian water, followed by spring water, and your last choice would be filtered water. Your goal should be a minimum of half your weight in ounces. So for a person who weighs 150 pounds, their goal is 75 ounces, or between four to five 16-ounce bottles of water.

Alcohol

This may get a little uncomfortable, but we have to address it, and I believe that this chapter is most ideal. Women are allowed one alcoholic beverage per day, ideally red wine, and men are allowed two servings. Now when you think of servings, I want you to think of the servings you get at a restaurant, not the large size beverages we get in Cancun or Las Vegas. This also does not mean you can save all your alcohol consumption for one day, meaning save your daily allowance for Saturday and have six drinks at one time. This is not beneficial to your health.

Chapter 9

To Snack or Not to Snack

I'm a snacker, a grazer as some would call it. Sometime my patients tell me they only eat 1-2 times a day because they're not hungry. I explain to them the reason they're not hungry is BECAUSE they are not eating. A little counter intuitive I know. Ever notice how when you skip breakfast you find that you're not hungry until lunch time, but if you eat breakfast, you're starving and can barely make it to lunch? That's because eating increases your metabolism. When you don't eat, your body goes into starvation mode and your metabolism slows down, which is why some patients can literally consume less than their required calories per day and not lose weight. Now the extreme opposite does not hold true. You cannot eat constantly and think you will lose weight. That precise balance is individual specific. Some individuals can eat three square meals a day, and that works well for their metabolism. Others require smaller meals with snacks throughout the day, and that is most ideal for their metabolism.

I found personally that when I only ate three meals a day, I was so hungry when it came time to the next meal that I would overeat. My lifestyle is very active, so on a daily basis I'm burning almost 2,000 calories a day. I found that three small meals with three snacks in between each meal works best for my metabolism. Dr. Powell, are you saying you eat six times a day?! That is exactly what I'm saying, and I would like to share with you some of my favorite go-to snacks.

Nuts: I always have a nut mix in my home. I purchase unsalted, natural, raw, no flavoring nuts. My favorites are almonds and pistachios. Make sure you yield to the serving size, because nuts do contain a lot of fat, albeit it is the good fats. Try to avoid the nut mix with salt or roasted with a flavor, because they often contain so much sodium! If you want to roast or add flavor to your nuts, you can easily do it yourself (with half the salt). Also try to avoid nut mixes with dried/dehydrated fruit because they can contain access sugar. I admit those dehydrated cranberries are my weakness. But be mindful that these contain extra sugar, so consume in moderation.

Fruit and/or vegetables with nut butter: This is another staple for me. I like to slice an apple or celery stick and eat it with peanut or almond butter. If I'm at home, I'll event sprinkle a little cinnamon on top. You can purchase nut butter in individual packets to make it easy on the go. This is a snack that adults and kids can enjoy.

Boiled eggs: This is also a go-to for me. On meal prep day, I like to boil six eggs and then have them to grab during the week—sometimes as an afternoon snack, other times as breakfast. If it's a meal like breakfast, I will eat two at a time. If it's an afternoon pick-me-up before the gym, I usually eat one. I sprinkle them with sea salt and cayenne pepper.

Smoothies: I have five signature smoothies that I keep in rotation based on what fruit and vegetables are in season. I can usually make five at a time, and between my husband and me, I replenish the supply every three days. Some smoothies are green, others protein-based, and then specialty ones made with Greek yogurt or iced coffee. Unless the smoothie has some kind of protein in them, they usually cannot supplement for an entire meal and are best as a snack or to complement a nice salad or sandwich.

Chapter 10

There's an App for That

In this day and age, you can pretty much assume that there is an app for whatever your health goals are, to make achieving those goals easier. I want to share with you some of my favorite apps that help me with my food and groceries, staying on track with my nutrition, and of course keeping up with my activity.

Instacart: This was a new one for me when I moved to Atlanta. Instacart allows you to access several grocery stores in your area, shop online, and have your groceries delivered in record time. You type your zip code in the app and they'll tell you what grocery stores you have access to. In my zip code, I have access to Publix, Costco, Aldi, and Whole Foods. There is a delivery fee, but this is also based on the time you select for your delivery. If you pick a popular time, it will be more expensive. If you have no delivery time requirements, then it's cheaper.

What I also like is your personal grocery shopper sends you updates as they're shopping. And if for whatever the reason the melons are not looking as fresh, they will send you an update and offer you an alternative. I love it and it definitely saves me time while I'm traveling.

Kroger: Kroger is one of my go-to grocery stores because of their prices. This is where, for the most part, I purchase our meat products. I like their app because I can shop online, get all the great Kroger deals, order my groceries, then select a time I plan on picking them up. So all my husband has to do is show up and pop the trunk. It's also nice for when I'm grocery shopping for my parents who live in a different state. I can order all their groceries, then they get a text message when they can come pick them up.

MyFitnessPal: This was an app I lived by in medical school and residency. When people tell me they're struggling to lose weight and are convinced it's not their diet because they "eat healthy," this is the first thing I ask them to do—download MyFitnessPal. This allows you to enter the food you're consuming throughout the day, and it adds up all the calories and nutrition information. Based on your age, current weight, ideal weight, and physical activity, it tells you how many calories you should be consuming on a daily basis. There is a barcode option, so you can scan the barcode of your food items, and the nutritional information loads automatically. What this app does essentially is create mindfulness. Now you are very much aware how much fat, protein, and calories you are consuming on a daily basis.

If you eat a high calorie breakfast and lunch then get to dinner and notice you only have 200 calories left until you reach your daily limit, you will be more mindful the next time about not consuming so many calories per meal. I had a patient who only ate fast food. She refused to cook any food. I asked her to download the app, continue to eat her fast food (which she refused to give up), and use the app daily. In two weeks, she lost seven pounds, still eating fast food. This was because she essentially became more mindful. She would see that at dinner time, she didn't have enough calories for the burger and fries, so she would not order fries. The app also allows you to add in your physical activity, which then increases the calories you can consume that day based on calories lost. So my patient was also motivated to do daily physical activity. Now my next step is to get her to cook one meal two days a week.

Yelp: Another app that I love (and that helps me with balance) is Yelp. You basically review user recommendations on all things food, shopping, night life, entertainment, restaurants, and things to do. Why's this important? Because it helps you plan. When it's date night, taking the in-laws out to dinner, or celebrating with the girls, it's important to have a list of go-to restaurants that you know will have menu items you can enjoy that stays within your health goals. I randomly search restaurants in my hometown and in cities I plan to visit so I can look for highly rated restaurants, review their menu, and see if there are options for me (vegetarian, low carb, not a plain vegetable platter, fresh high-quality seafood). I save those restaurants to a folder on the actual app. So I'm always prepared when a girlfriend calls me and says, " Let's go out to dinner. Where should we go?" I can raddle off a list of Dr. Powell-approved restaurants.

Chapter 11

Eating Healthily While Traveling

Travel should not be the thing that takes you off your game. Whether it's for work or pleasure, you have to be able to maintain your health goals while also being realistic. When planning your travel, I would like you to utilize the below checklist. Depending on the reason for travel, you may not have a say in this information, but many times you will at little to no additional cost.

- Does my hotel/villa/Airbnb have an exercise facility?

- Is safe to run around outside the hotel unaccompanied?

- Does my room have a refrigerator? If so, is there room to store your own personal food? So often I go to hotels and the fridge is full of for sale items and there's actually no room for me to store my own food.

- Is there a kitchen in my room?

- Is this an all-inclusive resort? If so, get a list of the restaurants and their menu.

- Are there any grocery stores nearby?

Knowing the above information allows you to do something critical: plan! Going on vacation is not what gets people off their regimen, because you can easily get off your regimen being at home. It's not having a plan that makes us fall off. If there is a local grocery store, before checking into your hotel, stop by and purchase some healthy snacks. Also purchase bottles of water, wheat bread, peanut butter and jelly for sandwiches, fresh fruit, veggies and humus, nuts, etc. If you have access to a kitchen, then you can also purchase things like eggs, oatmeal, black bean burgers, etc. To be able to make 1-2 of your daily meals will not only be better for staying on track but will also be a money saver.

We can't talk about travel without talking about...buffets. So I have two rules. First, just say no. The tendency with a buffet is to overeat. We get a little of everything as we walk through that line. We feel like since we paid for it, why not eat as much as possible? To order from the menu, as opposed to the buffet, is often not as good as a value as the buffet (i.e. a $20 all-you-can-eat breakfast buffet or an omelet for $17 and toast, sides, and coffee are extra). Even though the buffet is a better deal, I need you to plan on getting a plate instead if that's an option. Although you are paying more, you're doing what's best for your health. Now if there is no plate option, and you must partake in the buffet, this is how that process should work. Without a plate in your hand, I need you to walk through and survey the buffet. Look at all your options. Once you have done this, decide what your plate is going to look like and stick to the same rules you do at home and create a similar plate. You should not be eating some of everything. At home, you wouldn't make pancakes, omelets, waffles, a breakfast sandwich, fruit, a smoothie, a Danish, sausage, bacon, and ham. So don't make a plate of all this just because it is available to you. Be strategic.

Alcohol. This is where it gets a little tough for some. Especially with the all-inclusive resorts, it is tempting to consume as much as alcohol as you like.

I mean, why not? You've already paid for it. I'm going to be honest, during my all-inclusive honeymoon in Cancun, I definitely consumed more margaritas than food. My husband and I would wait for the bar to open at 11am and would end our evening with an 11pm margarita before bed. Let me tell you. When we returned from our honeymoon, I had gained half the weight I lost in preparing for our wedding, and this had significantly come from all the alcohol. Even though it's a beverage, it has calories. Try to limit your alcohol to one beverage a day. When you return home, your body will thank you.

Still try to exercise while on vacation, maybe even more! You're on vacation, which means you have more time. Start every day out with some exercise. Take advantage of classes at your hotel, the gym, or go for a run. When it's safe to do so and my husband allows, I love going for a morning run around town to find somewhere for us to eat breakfast.

Chapter 12

When Fast Food Is the Only Option

I was encouraged to write this chapter by my mentor. She is a physician, an entrepreneur, a mother, a wife, and she hates cooking! That's okay because she has a solution for juggling her busy life and not so strong relationship with the kitchen—a family chef. I don't think it gets much better than that, and even though I love to cook, I would love even more to have a chef do my cooking on those busy days where I just want to come home to a home-cooked meal. But for those times where she is traveling with her family, my mentor asked me what's the best and what to stay away from when it comes to fast food. And I think we should definitely talk about this. There will be unplanned times where you need to grab things quick and a local grocery store may not be an option. So I want to give you a list of things to say yes to and things to say no to.

Say No

- Anything fried

- Creamy dressings or sauce

- Super-sized anything (remember portion control)

- Sugary beverages (stick with water)

- Desserts, even if it's just an extra 0.99

- Two sandwiches for the price of one

Say Yes

- Salads (minus the croutons, bacon, and cheese)

- Grilled chicken

- Vinegar-based sauces and dressings

- Fresh fruit as a side

- A small fry (ask for no salt and add a little after)

- If you're going to have a sandwich, see if you can have large pieces of lettuce on the side (use these as buns). If this is not an option, use only one of the two pieces of bread.

- If the restaurant has healthy sides, get a few extras for later (I always get double of the kale salad from Chick-Fil-a)

Chapter 13

Sugar and Its Alternatives

I think it's super important that we discuss sugar. First, let's start with the basics. Sugar is metabolized to fats and carbohydrates which is why we do not want to mindlessly eat it. It's always better to use foods that are naturally sweet to sweeten up your food—fruit, dates, honey, and maple syrup to name a few. But it's important to note that all these sweet items are eventually broken down into glucose, which is the simplest form of sugar. This means that we still need to be mindful about how we utilize these items, particularly if you are someone who has a hard time metabolizing sugar, as seen in a diabetic. Below, I will list my top three favorite sugar substitutes.

Honey is my absolute fave! I use it on my pancakes, in my smoothies, in my coffee, and on my fruit. It is naturally sweet while also containing valuable nutrients. If you have the opportunity to purchase local honey, always go for it! Honey has medicinal purposes as well, which is why it's part of my home remedies for patients with a respiratory infection. Honey has anti-inflammatory, antibacterial, and antiseptic properties. It helps fight colds and ease cough symptoms. Now the downside to honey is that it does contain a fair amount of calories, so it still needs to be utilized in moderation.

My next fave is birch sugar, which is made from some fruits and vegetables, mostly corn due to the cost. It's crystals are larger than the standard sugar, which offers a nice texture to dishes. It is also low in calories, compared to honey and maple syrup. Longitudinal research on birch sugar is still underway, so long-term side effects and health benefits are still unknown.

Stevia is a sugar substitute that actually comes from a plant. A dear friend of my mother's actually grew the stevia rebaundiana plant species and would travel with stevia leaves, and this is what she would use to sweeten her tea. It is naturally very sweet, sweeter than sugar, so when converting between traditional sugar and stevia, equal parts cannot be used. It does not contain any nutrients.

Meal Prep Checklist

Meal prep has saved my life and has been key to being able to get so much done during the week while still eating clean. But to be honest, cooking for my myself and my husband—two people who eat very differently—for seven days can be overwhelming. So here are a few tips I use to streamline things. Note, I don't eat meat during the week and can eat the same thing every day. My husband eats lean meat and can't eat the same thing more than twice.

- Divide the week in half. On Sunday, prep for Mon-Wed, and on Wednesday, prep for Wed- Fri.

- For myself, I pick one grain (e.g. brown rice) and make a big pot and eat that every day as my starch. I switch grains each week.

- I always roast a tray of vegetables, and these can be repurposed for various meals.

- I boil some eggs for a quick-grab for breakfast or lunch.

- Pasta, made of legumes, is one of the staples in our house because I can usually get at least two meals out of it.

- Lunch for me is a bunch of vegetables that I chop in a bowl then put on a bed of whatever greens for a salad.

- For my husband, I focus more on prepping his dinner. Breakfast is usually cereal, and for lunch he buys a salad.

- Make smoothies on Sundays and freeze them. Put them in the refrigerator the night before to unthaw when you want to drink them.

Smoothie Secrets

I was a juicing queen back in residency! My fellow residents used to say that my juice looked like something found at the bottom of an ocean. Then I started making my green juice for my fellow residents and even my attendings. They loved them and never disrespected my smoothies again.

Juicing and making smoothies can be an excellent way to get more vegetables and fruits in your diet, but you still have to be mindful of the quantity of the ingredients you are using. I remember my dad telling me what he puts in his smoothies in the morning, and I said, "Dad, you're putting an entire fruit basket!" Plus, things like milk and yogurt adds extra calories. I'm all about keeping it simple. So when my patients tell me they want to make smoothies, I give them these basic principles when they are starting out:

- One vegetable, two fruits (1/2 each). I'll put as much spinach as I want, then do 1/2 banana and 1/2 apple.

- Use water for the liquid. You'd be surprised that it tastes just as good as adding milk or yogurt.

- Use honey for a sweetener.

- Juice of 1/2 lemon helps cut the earthy taste (lol).

- Use juicing/smoothies as an opportunity to get extra fiber, vitamins, minerals, and healthy fats by adding flaxseeds or chia seeds; they don't add any extra taste.

Simple Green Smoothie Recipe

This is my afternoon pick-me-up in clinic. Instead of having a second cup of coffee in the afternoon, I drink 16 ounces of this beauty and have the energy I need to power through the rest of my word day and my after-work workout.

Serves approx. two 16-ounce glasses

<u>Ingredients</u>
- 2 handfuls of spinach

- 200 mls of water (I like to use coconut water)

- 1 granny smith apple (really any yellow or green apple will do)

- 1 cup of strawberries

- 1 lemon

- 1 squeeze of local honey

- 1 tsp of chia seeds

Instructions:

In a blender, add spinach and water. Blend just to shred the spinach and make room in the blender. Then add the strawberries, the apple sliced and cored, a squeeze of honey, ½ cup of ice, one lemon juiced, and then add the chia seeds. Blend until well-blended. I usually listen to a Drake or Beyoncé song. After I've danced for about two minutes, it's ready to go!

Signature Protein Smoothie

This is my go-to smoothie when I'm short on time for breakfast. What I like about it is that it reminds me of strawberry ice cream. It's super simple to make and is essentially fail proof.

Serves two 16-ounce smoothies

Ingredients

- protein powder of your choice (select one with 150 calories or less, 20g of protein per serving and less than 3g of sugar per serving). Also make sure you actually like the flavor. I always go with a vanilla flavor.

- one ripe banana

- fresh or frozen strawberries (1.5 cups)

- 200 mL of unsweetened organic almond milk

- 1 tbsp peanut butter

- ½ tbsp steel cut oats

Instructions:

In a blender, pour almond milk to 200 ml line. Add banana, strawberries, peanut butter, steel cut oats, protein powder, and ½-1 cup of ice, depending if any of your fruit was frozen. Blend until smooth. You will need to make sure the steel cut oats are thoroughly blended; you will have to dance to the entire three minutes of the Beyoncé song. Enjoy!

Roasting Vegetables Made Easy

Roasting your veggies is super simple and pretty hard to screw up. Just toss the vegetables (Brussel sprouts and a sweet potato are my favorite combo) in olive oil, salt, and pepper. Lay flat on a baking sheet (with aluminum foil or parchment paper). Bake at 425 for about 40 minutes.

And that's it! You can add extra flavor by adding fresh garlic or cumin before baking. Also, I drizzled some balsamic vinegar for extra flavor.

Reference

American Family Physicians, June 1, 2018, volume 97, 11, " Diets for Health: Goals and Guidelines."

About the Author

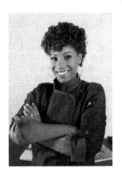

Lauren W. Powell, MD, is a board-certified family medicine physician and culinary medicine specialist. She received a bachelor's in chemistry and a minor in business from the University of Detroit Mercy. She later obtained her MD degree at Wayne State University School of Medicine and her family medicine residency at Halifax Health, where she was elected chief resident. During her residency, she presented several national research projects.

She furthered her training in culinary medicine at Tulane University School of Medicine to properly teach her patients about the role of food and health. Dr. Powell also served as a regular guest physician contributor on a radio show entitled *Healthy Living* with the mission of getting health-related information to minorities with limited access to the healthcare system. Her objective is empowering African Americans to end generational patterns of adverse health outcomes.

Follow her on social media @drlaurenpowell
and online at
www.DrLaurenPowell.com

CREATING DISTINCTIVE BOOKS
WITH INTENTIONAL RESULTS

We're a collaborative group of creative masterminds
with a mission to produce high-quality books to position
you for monumental success in the marketplace.

Our professional team of writers, editors, designers,
and marketing strategists work closely together to ensure
that every detail of your book is a clear representation
of the message in your writing.

Want to know more?
Write to us at info@publishyourgift.com
or call (888) 949-6228

Discover great books, exclusive offers, and more at
www.PublishYourGift.com

Connect with us on social media

@publishyourgift

CPSIA information can be obtained
at www.ICGtesting.com
Printed in the USA
FSHW011929130719